Walk Now

Live Forever

Viggo Pete Hansen

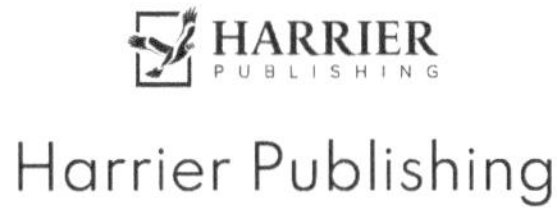

Harrier Publishing

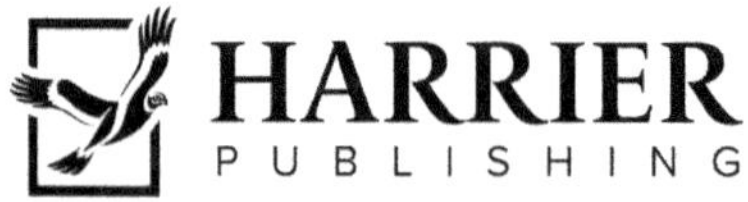

Published by Harrier Publishing

Tampa, Florida 33647 USA

www.harrierpublishing.com

Dedication

This book is dedicated to all who are now living and wish to live longer by walking regularly and - to those who will now faithfully take up a walking routine after reading this insightful document.

The initial inspiration for sharing my walking insights is due to Dixie Lee, my dearest life companion, who insisted on walking every morning beginning at 5 AM and - dragging me along. She then ran the first LA Marathon in her 40's and I am now following her inspiration in my mid- nineties.

VPH

Contents

Preface   VII

1. Life Is For Walking   1

2. Why Walk?   11

3. EVOLUTION of WALKING   14

4. Science of Walking   21

5. Categories of Walkers   27

6. Reminiscing   49

Preface

Truth Be Told!

<u>Absolutely nothing stands still – never has and never will.</u>

<u>So - walk today or atrophy tomorrow.</u>

Between what was and what will be lies our fleeting, illusive moment of what is, and that is being alive. "THE NOW - is THE WOW." Today is that glorious hot spot, where we always are – till we aren't. Life is defined by movement. Where and when there is no movement, there is no life. There is an expression for this: "all is gone". Be reminded as you luxuriate in your electronically controlled comfy bed, even while it is hot or cold outside,you still must move to stay alive. Lots of ideas here on what to do, especially getting up and going for a walk.

Our pitiful universe or maybe "multiverses" is/are seemingly indicating that we are going and getting somewhere to some unknown future. As the brilliant Webb telescope folks are expanding our understanding of what in heck went on in the past, just remember it was thinking walkers who got us this far, and will hopefully tell us where we may be headed.

Even rocks seem to get around, albeit slowly except when flying out of a burping volcano. Being stationary is anathema to all known Creators' prior designs – you gotta move to stay alive.

Walking, with feet, moving in any direction, is here understood as: Getting from A to B by use of original leg limbs and/or cleverly augmented prosthetic devices.

What is significant here is that the mind gets upset by inertness. Face it, your brain (however faulty the one you got is) is in charge of everything and abhors idleness. Brain is power.

There are variations on "walking" like; running, jogging, skipping, trotting, hopping, dancing, even crawling, slithering, and more. Still, the basic definition of walking remains: using your lower body parts, and adjuncts, in conjunction with your brain to get around and keep alive. If you think walking is dull and frivolous – please read on.

Like all historical events, walking has a murky beginning. Here is the current accepted version by this author. Many years ago, after the unknown big bang(s) , the brains of some bored unhappy swimmers in briney waters decided to experiment by wriggling around in unorthodox fashions. Hot, sunny days were problematic for living in the primordial swamps.

Thus, more creative thinking was needed to improve on using mud caked fins to get around. Furthermore, their muddied orifices led to unhappy egg-laying schedules, especially when the moon was not in optimum alignment. So they figured it was time to move from a dull, murky salty environment to a more compatible grassy area.

Ah ha - this was to become yet another evolutionary leap in the saga of "life", which of course we still have no idea what it really is. A lot of research is still needed here to fill in the unknown evolutionary gaps. Since "life" seems to be continually evolving it is essential that we learn from our foreparents to where we are headed, especially now that our legs may atrophy for lack of use.

Ergo: what is now going on with this waning of walking business is significant for predicting the evolution of "life".

Walking evolved just like everything else, this bumpity bump is similar to asteroids kicking our planet Earth around. Nature constantly makes alterations, always trying to overlook past booboos and keep seeking perfection – we hope. Question is, can we humans evolve out of our present existence by non-walking behavior? If they can and do - then what?

A related aside: Currently, there are some serious concerns about homo sapiens' political/religious ambitions and behaviors that will for sure affect their long-term evolutionary survival. Really, it is truly bewildering why we became – and remain – more interested in eradicating each other than in solving "stay alive" issues that support bettering eternal evolutionary trends for us all. Again, it seems clear that the more we walk and think good thoughts the better the chances of our survival become.

So for the moment let us leave the philosophical, political discussions somewhere else and focus on the exciting walking issues, which we can do something about.

If everything had remained stationary, i.e., no evolution, we would long ago have reached perfection – as rocks have. Imagine, just lying there quietly basking in sunshine with soft flowing waters running over you - forever. No way would this satisfy our restless brains. Instead; consider no pollution, no politics and religions and with endless opportunities for creative activities, and of course - hiking.

What is more exciting than a John Philip Sousa marching band energizing kids and adults alike, as they briskly parade triumphantly up and down Main Streets of our world? These are the survivalists, while the standby non-walkers, mostly politicians, are yapping about how to spend your money.

This book is all about the marvelous and essential experiences of walking, its health values and personal enjoyments with near zero cost factors. It also opens the door to questions about where human evolution is headed?

The future for walking is unknown and possibly bleak, judging by the increasing size of humans who sit on their gluteus maximus most of the time. As many now shun walking, industries see opportunities to enhance their bottom lines by creating ever bigger wheels and devices needed to get us about. As our legs may slowly atrophy for lack of use, just like the fins became legs on certain bygone fish years ago, we now might begin sprouting biological type wheels, bigger butts, and strange appendages to hold eye-level cell phones, along with raven-like wings for soaring. Yes, this is exciting stuff, eh? And all because we gave up walking.

Oh my goodness, no knee and hip replacements will be necessary, since they will have atrophied. Old body parts inflicted with arthritis and other debilitating ills will be phased out. Other bodily functions related to walking will also evolve.

For instance; when walking, eyes are busily focusing all over the place and sending information to the brain.

In the future, When not walking and focusing on a computer screen, eyeballs will probably evolve to accommodate large rectangular flat screens. Sound will be provided by some kind of gizmo that will filter out random sounds now enjoyed when walking. We will be deprived of birds tweeting, kids yelling, bloody auto crashes, emergency sirens and weird flying objects. And for gosh sake don't overlook the variety of wondrous smells that walks abundantly experience, you know - what in the world is that smell?

In many ways when giving up walking the future seems to be drifting towards control using eyeballs and fingers to go anywhere and get things done. But let us never overlook the fact that it is our brains that are in charge. What our brain wants – our brain gets, including the desire to walk and live longer. Major question? What is the brain up to? Artificial Intelligence suggests perhaps brains are evolving in truly unknown ways.

Recap:

FINS WERE FOR SWIMMING.

LEGS FOR WALKING.

BEHINDS FOR SITTING.

FINGERS FOR TEXTING.

WILL EYEBALLS SOON DO IT ALL?

AND THEN WHAT?

BRAIN ONLY!

Be aware – this book is heavy stuff.

It is all about YOUR life!

Chapter One

Life Is For Walking

There appears to be a strong connection between any "living" organism and its "mind." Some might argue for the hierarchy "mind over body (matter)," but that can certainly be challenged on many levels. A mind with no body is as useless as a body with no mind. To be safe let us agree that mind and body depend on each other for mutual survival. Furthermore, if either doesn't survive, they both quickly expire.

Today, wonderful walking trails are everywhere, globally, from your backyard, to your local shopping mall, to magnificent mountains. They are perhaps the best resource for humans to do great thinking and to live longer. Some walks are done by groupies (two or more), but perhaps the most benefited walkers are those who walk alone. This is not meant to disparage "yakker" walkers. Their bodies will still benefit, but as for mental benefits, we have no researched supportive evidence.

Walking is ubiquitous. For many it begins in the morning by going from bed to bathroom and ends at night by going from bathroom back to bed. Too often the interval between these daily mini-treks are impaired by stressful thinking. In the AM, it is: What I am going to do today to be free of (Fill in your own blank, e.g. potential jail time, divorce, kids flunking grades, heart attack). By PM, What was this day all about?

But hark! Just remember that every step taken that day was a step to know yourself better, and wow - you will now also live longer. (only to do it all over and over again for a longer time . . . hmm.) Psychologically this technique is known as "Walking Stress Away." An aside: There are of course cynics who misinterpret this as walking for more misery.

The path currently pursued by many humans, i.e., sitting and staring at screens while finger-tapping, may be the beginning of an entirely new evolutionary era. Animal ontogeny has moved from conception to swimming to crawling to walking and now - who knows what lies ahead?

Effortless exercises with expensive gadgets and the lack of walking may not augur well for maintaining our current species' mind and physique. The evolutionary path from fish to swarthy toads and frogs to the erectus human status happened very slowly as life as we know it today began. We are now physically somewhat out of the muck, but have mentally strayed into an uncharted quagmire of taking it easy in recliners, drinking a variety of human made liquids and complaining about most everything. These behaviors are totally incompatible with old time walking.

This leads to the question of what kinds of movements are best suited for mind/body growth, longevity and personal happiness. Sure enough, evolution has now produced a variety of industries ranging from gurus in technology loaded spas to love boat tours and mountain top chalets; just like fish of old, we are all continuing seeking alternative lifestyles. No kid wants to sit still - but with age some have perfected unbelievable sit-down skills, seeking and finding many paths and trails to a walkless/lying down nirvana; sort of reminding us of fish.

The "Walking Away Stress Movement" is based solely on getting one's behind off flat surfaces and putting attached legs into a swinging motion, called "gait", a motion most humans are generously endowed with from early childhood.

When walking, the ever-controlling mind is given a break from debilitating human-made computer stresses and given freedom to rejuvenate life and recover its innate god-given creativity.

Background: Early on, evolutionarily speaking, moving about by swimming was the only option for our ancestor fish, who at that time were the primary animals in existence on this planet. Plant evolution is something else not covered here.

But of course swimming got quite boring to some restless teenage fish, called teeny bob fishes. Puberty for all animals is a turbulent time. The first shedding of scales when growing into fish adulthood is stressful. Mommy and Daddy-O fish were clueless regarding what to do with their teenagers.

Something had to be done. Adult fish, though confused by their youthful progeny's unconventional behavior, were aghast but they were probably also envious (like most parents today). Older parent fish worried evolution was passing them by. They sensed that a scaleless, hip-swinging Elvis was in the fantasized unattainable future. Little did they suspect that AI (artificial intelligence) was also coming down the pike. Every step in the evolutionary chain of events is a surprise.

Recapping: From egg and sperm making whoopee to becoming a spiny, scaly fish was exhilarating. The evolutionary phases that followed were unpredictable and thrilling. Ever so slowly the upstart rebellious youth have again and again led us to the brink and into another new lifeform. Today we walk less, finger poke/swipe more, and rightfully stress about where we are headed. Solution to our stress: Walk more.

Lots of birthdays, exhilarating trips around the sun, all in a cosmic realm poorly understood, are still taking place, as we "humans" continue to evolve. Life's rambunctious brains are always on the move to find something new and different. When will our legs atrophy and become useless? Perhaps soon, if we don't use them. Maybe that is how evolution really works. Use it or lose it. Perhaps we are now in a time of transitioning.

While some of us believe that human evolution began at a fishy stage, there might also have been, or are, other subatomic stages, or even non-atomic stuff going on. Walking, while thinking about evolution, might just open the door to a vision of the future – maybe a renaissance from physical to mental.

While various life forms have taken up flying (birds), and some, like fish, have remained in the ocean, somehow humans became walkers. Plants, rocks, and stars have their own evolutionary histories, but we humanoids have drifted into upright physical bipeds following our stint as slimy, venturesome creatures frolicking on muddy beaches.

There are lots of really serious philosophical and religious versions of our evolutionary trajectory that have too often led to nasty behaviors called politics, wars, and pollution. These activities, including scientific understanding, may indeed alter our otherwise natural evolutionary progression. Are we, by not walking, modifying where we were otherwise naturally headed? Are today's walkers, or non-walkers, determining the future? Think about that as you sit on your duff tapping incredible devices. You may be a futurist with a short lifespan – while walkers enjoy a happy long-term existence.

Evolutionary events are truly revolutionary. Once erstwhile uppity fish got acclimated on land, they saw many new possibilities. They were oh, so happy. That is why fish, to this very day, look like they are smiling, just like many of today's walkers. Walkers are also smilers.

Yes, today walking is so gratifying. Early on humans sensed that walking was to be the future. From swimming to slithering, creeping, crawling, and finally walking. Walking became a truly great new existence. Every step taken was historical, based on past experiences,all with an expanded positive view of a better future. Caveat: This was true until lawyers invented politics.

As my biology professor said, "Ontogeny recapitulates Phylogeny." This sort of means that we humans, early on as we matured, may have experienced the many exciting evolutionary life stages that preceded us, including sperm swimming while merrily chasing cute ova. Wowie. Today this activity is known by many adults as a dating service adventure leading to bliss and the happiness of getting a gorgeous, squealing bundle of joy at three AM. This recapitulation concept is certainly a very clever scientific observation by biologists and a really fun topic for philosophers, gurus, preachers, heavy thinkers, and drinkers to pursue while on leave from menial tasks.

The evolution of human foot movements may be viewed as a natural progression of nature. Swimming, using lots of movements, similar to flying, is pretty much three-dimensional. One can swim in all directions, up, down, and sideways. Walking, however, may be viewed as simply a two-dimensional activity: back and forth. Going up and down stairs hardly qualifies for three-dimensional status. Furthermore, two-legged walking is quite a unique activity. Even chickens know and appreciate this.

So what comes next? Based on the findings of these independent in-depth investigations, which are totally based on simple observations and with no government funded research, we can safely opine "we don't know," and most don't give a hoot. While many enlightened folks may not take walking too seriously, just remember: If you walk a lot now, you may just live a lot longer.

Furthermore, maybe our next evolutionary walk will be one of timelessness. Won't that be great? Just think – walking back and forth without being restricted by time (whatever time is). This will become the new age of "the Eternal Hike." Better get ready for the future by practicing today.

Another exciting potential of walking in the future has to do with quantum notions, like possibly walking in two places at the same time – just as the electrons that make up the atoms that make up our bodies seem to do. The human mind remains restless, seeking new opportunities built on walking skills.

Hopefully without physical and mental pain, we may anticipate that our species is about to make a major futuristic leap from physical use of legs to an emphasis on pure mental walking. Again we are reminded that today's walking with legs is controlled by the ever-present mind. If the mind doesn't need to fuss with legs, just imagine the possible places to go and activities to do!

Summary: Walking evolved when some rebellious fish left the primordial swamp, a long time ago of course, to slither, slide, then crawl, and finally walk. Fascinating how today walking is again evolving (or is it devolving), making our legs obsolete. As our bodies get bigger, we humans rely more on wheels and other contraptions instead of walking to get from A to B. This is probably not good for prolonging the current status.

Now comes some exhilarating "breaking news." As folks today give up walking and gain lots of kilos, we are witnessing the public relations power of the non-walkers. This avant-garde movement is enthusiastically fueled by the wheel makers, energy companies, and cellphone enthusiasts. The arising routine is: drive, yell, sit, but for sure don't walk.

Are we perhaps seeing the rise of a new non-walking "human being"? Just look around.

This book is a must-read for everyone who wants to live longer and might be interested in preserving the historical nature of walking by seeking more information on why and how we should. The kicker here is that leg-walkers are ideally adaptable for the future mind-walkers. Remember, it is always your restless mind that makes the first moves.

Walking is the essence of living mentally. If you were lucky enough to have gotten a brain, you are endowed with the ability to walk, at least mentally. Everyone can enjoy and appreciate the wonderful "art of walking" regardless of age, daily trivia, and the nincompoops cluttering up your life.

Those of us with physical handicaps now have a variety of support systems that allow our bodies to sense and dream of being in walking motion. The extent that our "walking thoughts" may influence our mental and physical lives is a personal matter – but we know the influence is great. And great physical therapists are available to facilitate this benefit.

It has got to be sad for those who need help walking to witness those who can walk, but needlessly use vehicles that pollute the atmosphere for us all. This comment is to make non-walkers feel guilty and ashamed.

All kinds of statistics and generalized baloney, in all kinds of media, are readily available regarding this business called walking. We recommend ignoring all of them. Ignore the meaningless chatter on how to walk, what to wear, proper cuss words to use, and where to walk. All that is legally needed is to cover your private parts and then just walk, inside or outside, and have a few yucks along the trail(s). Your body will thank you by extending your current "alive" time, and perhaps even prepare you for an unknown eternal time.

Historical Recap:

It surely must have been amazing to watch, when years ago, a bunch of nonconformist teenage fish, who had finally gotten sick and tired of swamp life (similar to today's computer nerds), somehow came up with the unconventional concept of taking a stroll on dry dirt. Except for the unicorns, fish had pretty much been moving around horizontally. But once on land, exposing too much of their belly to rough terrain became a pain.

This historical evolution of life, poorly documented, that began eons ago, is now interestingly enough quite similar to today's restless teens who – with their wheels of all descriptions, selfies, eyes glued to screens, and wires stuck in their ears – are now yearning for new vistas, etc. They, too, are pioneering a new way on the evolutionary tree of life to a new world, just like the fish of old.

Fingers and eyeballs are indeed now beginning to replace legs, just as legs replaced the fins of yore. The really spooky future may have to do with what comes after the current brain is replaced by "AI " - artificial intelligence? Did the now questionable "Big Bang" theory include infinite evolutionary stages? Now the buzz is artificial intelligence. Does anyone really know what intelligence really is? This is teehee stuff and calls for another round of favorite libations, even warm milk..

Human Evlution

After love making

Swimming

On to crawling

Then walking

Today texting.

Then what ?

Eyeballing?

Artificial Intelligence?

MENTAL TELEPATHY?

Weird Drawing

May whatever gods there be better help us all.

Artificial Intelligence?

MENTAL TELEPATHY?

Weird Drawing

Chapter Two

Why Walk?

S imply to get from A to Z. To your ATM. To the bar. To the bathroom and back to the bar. These and other significant reasons suffice to understand why we depend on walking. But perhaps the most important reason to walk is to better get to know yourself in your environment and extend your life on this planet. If you really want to.

The previous chapter on how walking may have begun is maybe "swampy" silly and quasi-factual speculation. Today, people like you and me didn't just wake up and start walking with smiling faces, swinging arms, singing happy lilts or mouthing chatter, all while praying not to be hit by a meteor. No,no! Our ability to do this means each one of us has luckily lived through the many evolutionary stages of our phylum, from fishlike sperm to finally becoming today's healthy, erect, jolly walkers.

Question: Just who are today's walkers?

Answer: The restless vagabonds, just like the fish and toads that preceded us.

We now recognize that the walking phenomenon has had a fascinating bit of evolutionary history. For some walking is pretty boring stuff, while for others it is refreshing, exhilarating, and life-extending. For the minimal walkers, their physical activity, while watching their favorite sports team on a comfy couch, consists of limping to the refrigerator for a cool one and verbally expressing dissatisfaction with their team's loss.

Let us ponder on how walking, now taken for granted by many, is tragically also ignored by many humans. Here comes heavy stuff to ponder. Is the demise of walking the precursor of the next evolutionary stage? As mentioned earlier, have we perhaps begun to evolve into a new lifeform?

This evolutionary trend may be an omen of what our species may be doing in future eons. Relying on misinformation and dusted with fantasy thinking, we may have the wonderful opportunity to predict our future. This all depends on what we do with our turbulent present.

The fantastic good news is that those who continue to walk are living longer and may actually become futurists.

Young-uns can't wait to walk. They struggle mightily to stand on two feet, and once they know how to ambulate, there is no stopping them. They are underfoot everywhere. But today the trend is to give these upstarts a soft chair and devices that emphasize using eyeballs and fingers (no wonder they are called digital!), not legs. Staring at screens, tapping and swiping with fingers, and racing wheeled vehicles are definitely in – all generously supported by hi-tech industries and, of course, parents, teachers, politicians, and religious gurus. Fish and toads were more limited in options.

That is until they became "human." Now, interestingly enough, many who are not sports-minded have devolved to again being fishlike, lying horizontally most of the time and using only their thumbs and fingers for movement and communication. With eyeballs glued to the movement of mischievously clever icons on media screens, they make few movements in their bodies. Legs are used sparingly, except maybe for decorations and buying rarely used walking shoes.

Is this not exciting? You bet, we may be seeing a new modified species. Evolution never stops - Whoopee

Chapter Three

EVOLUTION of WALKING

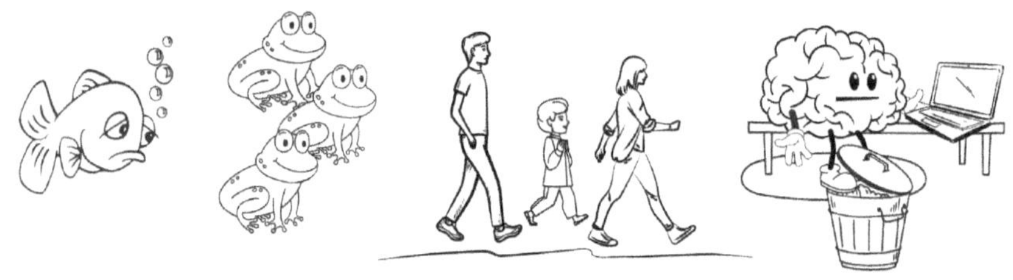

Evolution of Walkers

Flash back to the beginning of our ancestors' life in a saline environment. It was probably some bluish liberal-thinking fish youngsters who finally admitted they were bored out of their existence. They had no cute underwater cheerleading soccer fish, with bull horns and acrobatic routines, encouraging teams to get in the net. So, tired of aimless swimming with eely family members, eating mostly kelp salads without dressings, and bigger fish chewing away on them, they began looking for a new life. They agreed there must be a safer and better dining place.

These unhappy beady-eyed lifeforms had to be restless and finicky. They probably wondered if there might not be a more exciting way to get around and conjure up some new games. However, some did have reservations about losing their current three-dimensional swimming capabilities.

Finally, one cloudy day – which all underwater days were and are – these cranky, hormonal, acme-scaled and -pocked fishies rebelled. The evolutionary calendar began. You know the kind of folk. Today they drink a lot of fortified coffee and/or other adult beverages, then decide to put biology on a new and more creative path forever.

Restless fishy genes got busy. The past was past. We must now move ashore and become toadlike.

These liberal minded fish now did become early toad upstarts. They had had enough of the existing creationism mentality. We must evolve. Whoever was responsible for what life had become in the ocean, that lifestyle now needed a more uplifting and cultured revision. Swimming had gotten boring. Furthermore, big fish eating little fish remained an evolutionary issue. Interestingly enough, today it is big companies eating little ones.

"Let us go a-swamping" became the go-to daily slogan.

In summary, life in the briny was awful, tasted bad, made for an all over itch and it reeked. Kiddy toads could easily evade parents by slithering away, making childhood discipline and education impossible. The entire kit and caboodle of toad life lifestyle needed overhaul – or - try to create an entirely modified life form. Ergo, another evolution. Toads, at least some uppity ones, now wanted to be called frogs. They thought, "Why must we surface to take a breath of fresh air? Why not get out of this slippery stuff, and walk upright like – like what? Let us call them 'walking animals' - later to become nicknamed "humans".

This was a time in history when the National Fish Evolution Association (NFEA) was born. Their mantra: "We have the evolutionary right to get out of the swamp and protect ourselves." Now here is a caveat. Today there are some humans who see this as the beginning of democracy. If the government is imperfect, blame the fish constitution. If you are a fourth/fifth grade teacher or parent of one,, you know exactly the kind of "fish" we are referring to (not your kid, of course).

So one dreary morning millions of years ago, before BCE and AD were in vogue, some zit-infected fish skipped his early morning AP class on "gill-flossing" (a very smart fish), thinking life is too short for this inane gill health nonsense and rebelled. A new life form began.

You know how smart teen kids can be. An alpha macho (John Wayne) fish swam close to the beach and used his fins to slither up on Miami's, or with luck Rio's, beautiful sandy beach. This unorthodox male fish (it is always males that cause trouble), thought he had died and gone to fish heaven. Unbelievable. He exploded with joy from his wet dream and quickly slithered/swam back and convinced his Advanced AP Gill Floss classmates to join him exploring a glorious new frontier on land.

With some bullying efforts he did get a congregation of venturesome colleagues to follow. Up on the sandy, crab-infested beach they crawled, absolutely fish-eyed at what they saw. Oh yes, the female fish immediately wanted to know where to get dental floss bikinis. Much better use of floss than on one's gills. Oh, no! Evolution has taken a new step somewhere.

A major concern at this point in evolution was the business of spawning, i.e., keeping the ole family tree a-growing. You can just bet this was tricky, as these adventuresome young critters, historically used to lovemaking in the mud, now had to conjure up more creative techniques. But again creativity and experimentation provided solutions. Life will win out as always.

Spawnology counseling took a big leap upward and became a much sought-after career objective. No more long treks in the ole swamp, eh? Fish gurus of the time began looking for techniques and chemicals to enhance the procedure of mud spawning without getting mired down in mud. Their bestseller of that time was nicknamed and marketed as "Mud-up." The next stage from mud to human erectus is pure speculation, so it will not be discussed here.

This concludes the somewhat willy-nilly history of men's and women's early ventures into replacing swimming in the mud with walking on the beach. This is not to disparage those who must have their mud baths, however. These folks simply have stronger memories of their evolutionary trek.

Walking is an ideal movement condition: upright body in synchronous motion, autonomic systems balanced, and burning calories while leaving the almighty brain free to meander in its imaginative and creative universe, spun of the myriads of grayish neurons that comprise what we loftily call our mind and define who we are. It is easy to imagine the many opportunities for nefarious mischief in this arrangement. It probably accounts for why many insecure folks fail to walk: They are scared.

However, there are many places in our world – lots of them – where to get anywhere you have to walk. Interestingly, here you find fewer insecure people, fewer on sugar-free and low-fat diets, and much less polluted air. They are too busy looking for shoes.

For those who, sadly, cannot walk as they wish, there are "thought and memory walks" whereby your mind multitasks by imagining the real thing. No physical distractions, just you the mind walker and your memory, enjoying mental visions of moving through our incredible universe. Some of humankind's greatest thinkers have and are mental (not physical) walkers. They may be the ultimate "walkers." Stephen Hawking comes to mind.

From here on the "Walker Story" becomes really exciting, yet murky. It's fascinating how our earlier Homo sapiens buddies finally got to where we all are today, especially how we all developed different religions, skin colors, and politics. Was it the damn fish, who didn't all come from the same swamp? You really have to ponder on their religious/political affiliations as evolution keeps trying to make us all happy – and a place to go when this doesn't all work out. For sure, "Evolvers" look forward to happy hour every day – some with a bit of a kick, others more soberly with a spot of tea. But what the heck. Fish were finally up and walking about.

There exists an enchanting history on how philosophical topics were discussed while walking woodland trails – all over the world. Often these thinkers walked with their hands behind their back. Probably not recommended by modern orthopedists; but if it makes one feel good – do it.

A conjecture could be made that if political office seekers discussed controversial issues while walking steep mountain trails in the dead of night, they would come up with some significant ideas. If all leaders and managers would go walking in the woods and learn to think before they talk, they might say some sensible and clever things. You know, "Walk your talk."

Today too many of us have stuff constantly going into our heads via a variety of distracting gizmos instead of internally conjuring up our own creative solutions. Everything is going in and little of importance is coming out. Mental slavery.

How about having politicians debate while walking. You would wonder how many could stay on topic and maintain cadence. Sure as hell might scare all the animals about them, including other human beings.

As we will now know, walking is great for the body, mind, and soul, but there are now impediments to personal physical and mental improvements. Earbuds, smart/mostly dumb phones, tight-fitting butt-enhancing panties and shorts, and the like can and may often deprive today's walkers of personal benefits. That is why the walkers of old did it in the woods – walking, that is.

When using these distracting amenities, walkers are not learning and appreciating the external and internal world about them – by themselves. Mentally they probably don't even know they are walking. They are simply tapping and swiping and yakking like they usually do most of the time.

You have to wonder how many of the world's great/greatest ideas and creations were mentally conceived while their creator was walking. Primitive walking-thinking behavior, with no apps, are highly creative because they are so "you."

Walking brings new insights enhanced with memories of past experiences, creating new vistas and promises for the future. What helps make the walking experience so rich and vibrant are the unique varieties of sensations walkers encounter. Every sense organ, sight, smell, feel, and sound is stimulated and interwoven in the human mind.

Chapter Four

Science of Walking

This is the technical chapter on walking. It is somewhat heavy stuff and can easily be omitted if you are short on time or bored by science. If need be, go see your doctor, but she/he is probably on the golf course practicing walking and hopefully not riding a buggy.

Walking depends on two powerful forces: one, physical stuff like gravity and muscles, but more importantly, two: it is the human mental attitude – you know, mind over matter – that counts.

Step One.

First, before beginning to walk, you must get yourself into a mental frame of mind. Easy on non-water libations, This is absolutely critical. Once your mind is ready, your body will, as always, follow instructions. You now get out of bed, or off a recliner chair, and stand up erect – with a smiling, determined look. Lazy folks around you may feel intimidated by your demeanor. You will now look like a victorious Napoleon after getting off his horse, without falling, and smirking about having conquered something.

If you think this is tough for you, just be reminded how, early on, the poor determined fish struggled to get out of the swamp and into the mud. Today we humans can be thankful we do not have this same challenge in common with guppies, koi, barracuda, and orcas. For the sake of brevity we will overlook frogs and toads and skip to erect humans.

Step Two.

Gravity is constantly fighting you for your entire life span on our planet and especially while you walk. Gravity is well understood, to the point where there are now clever formulas showing how it all works out and keeps everything from flying every which way – or not moving at all. Newton's ripe apple tree helped him create equations to explain why apples fell in his day and still fall today, many years later. Luckily, oday's walkers don't need to sit under an apple tree to understand this physics stuff in order to be proficient and long-living walkers. Just do it..

It is gravity that keeps us all close to the earth. For example, when you lift a leg and plan to move it forward, it is gravity that pulls it back to the ground. You really have to work at overcoming the earth's gravitational attraction for you.

Gravity's wish is to have everything, us included, come to squat in the center of the earth. That is just the earth's gravity – but golly gee, there are also many other gravitational forces tugging at us. The sun and moon come to mind.

Now, when we come to those powerful forces called human desire, emotions, and intents, all bets are off. Scientists have for years tried to write equations regarding people's whims with absolutely no success. What they do know for a fact is that people will walk, but only if they want to walk or are really scared. Conversely, if they don't want to walk, they probably won't, barring a terrific incentive. Bottom line is – people will walk only if they can and want to do it. Psychology is great, eh? Ego wins. We do know that with the help of gravity, walking is theoretically possible and actually done by billions of people on a daily basis because they have to make a buck.

But wait! The apparatus needed for walking is also part of the overall scheme of universal walking principles. You need legs and feet (real or artificial), and a connected torso all loaded with itty-bitty and huge bones. All of these pieces have Latin names if you are of European descent. Other names are used by other nationalities, but they all mean the same thing.

Bones are hard and in general will not bend a whole lot, so a bunch of them can function (move) by using slippery stuff between them, just like WD-40 on door hinges to the bathroom, so no one knows where you are going, eh? Bones need the same kind of fragrance-free lubricant so you don't sound like Oz's Tin Man.

An aside. It is interesting that humans have bones for structure, but fish have a different structural arrangement, allowing them to float. Herein lies another mystery: just how did the adventurous swamp fish change their bones and attachments to walking upright? Probably slowly.

Humans on average begin at birth with some 270 bones, provided they are not short-changed at conception, during delivery, or by accident. By adulthood (for those that make it) something has happened, and they have only about 206 left. But you know what?

Many, many of these bones, big and tiny, are somehow used for walking. For example, the pinky toe is attached to the upper leg bone, a big sucker called the femur, which then is attached to the torso at the pelvic bone. Stuff for poets and songwriters.

When humans walk they of course use all their leg bones and also tend to swing their arms for balance. Then the neck bones adjust the head for optical scanning so you can see to avoid colliding with anything or worse somebody.

This is getting technical, but please hang in there. Again all these bones, from the femur to the tiny bone at the end of the little-piggy toe, are elegantly and efficiently hitched together with the brain to enable moving synchronously in what is commonly referred to as walking. There you have it. Furthermore, walking can be richly enhanced by variations like running, jumping, skipping, or hopping. Stretching these activities into a watery environment, they are technically called swimming, reminiscent of our fishy/toady forebears.

Now comes the need for a power source to move all these bones in response to the mental messages coming from the brain's ego: "I want to go somewhere." This incredible power source, we call muscle. Muscles are remarkable. They push and pull things by telling, directing, and orchestrating the movement of legs, arms, gall bladders, and heads when suggested by the walker's mind – which is always suspect of its motives.

You may now understand where this is going. To live longer, you must walk longer, but all this wonderfulness depends on attitudes. Ergo, walking is an attitude.

It's fascinating to realize that after the fish became walkers, they created a whole bunch of sporting activities, from tiddlywinks to banging each other's head with their fists in all kinds of games. Observers of these events make and lose money betting on outcomes. And boy, oh boy, did these activities provide research opportunities and sustenance for medically smart folks. Modified walking games, sports, and wars became a money-maker.

To summarize: Walking involves a mindset capable of orchestrating moving parts: femurs, tibias, fibulas, patellas, teeny toe bones, cartilage, tendons, ligaments, and so much more. This is not trivial. It means that walking is, in scientific terms, damn tricky and maybe at times irritating, while also prolonging life.

To fully understand and appreciate this medical stuff on walking, always consult with your doctor about authenticity or read the countless materials available. Personal testimonials regarding veggies, especially rutabagas, are titling technical stuff but fun to read but pretty useless. Disclaimer: no reputable doctors are contributing to the author's scientific walking biases, his whereabouts, or mental status.

Chapter Five

Categories of Walkers

Not only is it fun, educational, and informative to watch walkers walk, but it can also be enlightening. Just like Charles Darwin, you, too, can witness various stages of an animal's walking evolution. Like all animals seen in the Galapagos Islands or Manhattan streets and around the planet, each species is unabashedly expressing its private journey through eons of nature's wonderful evolutionary designs – even many that didn't work out so well. Why, oh, did we lose those beautiful unicorns?

But there is more to the theory of walking style. Each one of us walks differently. This is another example of how the universe "Maker(s)" has a foolproof defense. Every one of us is unique, based on the premise to never make the same mistake twice. So, since we are all different, our walking is as different as our thinking.

Since walking in public, or privately, is pretty much unregulated and also guaranteed by all inalienable rights and amendments promised by political folks, it is an expression of our divinely bestowed freedoms. However, for what it is worth now, walking was not legally guaranteed by our founders who conjured up the US Constitution. Be aware that non-walker fringe groups may be shortening our average life expectancy.

If you have a lot of data, from watching and participating in walking, you can create an infinite number of categories, one for each unique walker. To assist in understanding this concept, we have simplified your life by making broad categories. These are just a guide to better appreciate and simplify the complexity of, and respect for, each walker's individuality. Again: "Our Gods never make mistakes twice; they created each of us really, really different."

CATEGORIES

A. Thinking Walkers

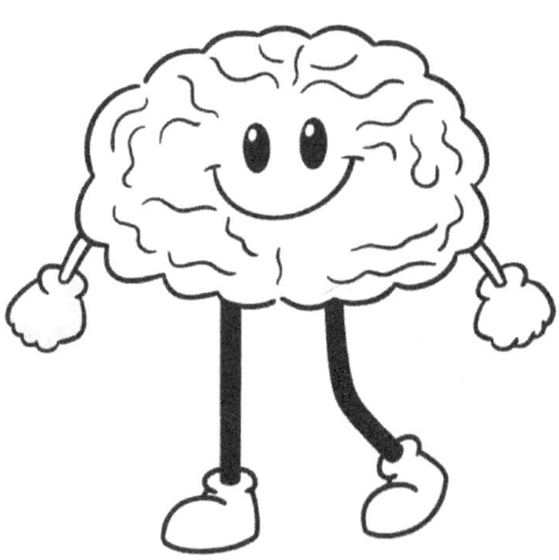

Thinker walkers were, are, and will be the admired professional walkers of the past, present, and future. They wrestle with the deepest philosophical inner workings of the universe. Who, how, why, what, when, and where is the entire human life shebang headed? Heady stuff indeed.

Often these quiet folks amble along at their own thoughtful pace, deep into psychology, enjoying the ambiance of their personal moment, and oblivious of everyone else; true "be here now" existentialists. Their roots go back to antiquity, just like when fish swam out of the swamp.

A subcategory of these walkers are the dreamers, who have worked this personal metaphysical treat into their personal walking schedule and allow no one to interfere. This is their private time. Outwardly they have a lot in common with the thinker walkers, except they are perhaps more of the dreamy type. Some are very artistic, creating symphonies, novels, and what to eat for dinner as they extend their life by walking.

These are the true mind-body walkers, in full control of their lifestyle at this moment as they appreciate the gift of personal privacy. For the moment it is just them in their unique universe. Here is where creative ideas are born while simultaneously physical fitness is renewed.

Euclid, perhaps the greatest geometer of all time, concluded as a walker that his axioms would work a whole lot better if the world was flat, ergo plane geometry. Truth is that our earth is not a flat surface, and we must look out for potholes, mad dogs, and poorly behaved children.

Zeno's paradoxes constantly tease thinker walkers about how nobody is going anywhere because they can't get started. The business of convergence and divergence is fun to ponder. Just being content standing still is, of course, wonderful thinking to bona fide non-walkers. But this is naturally blasphemy to the antsy folks who wish to romp around in the bush, thinking they are going somewhere.

Throughout history pesky issues like determinism versus indeterminism have also needled many of these deep thinker walkers. In summary, their thoughts went something like this: What was, was; what it is, is; and what will be, will be. So is there free will, or are we simply someone's cosmic toy robots? Sadly, these kinds of thoughts may lead to excessive lust for liquids, thereby simultaneously creating new philosophies and religions.

While this stuff may seem quite rational to some, there were those walkers who maintained that just maybe what was, wasn't; what is, isn't; and what will be, won't be. There may be observational data that the more walkers think about this, the faster they move.

This conundrum is what kept the walkers-of-old hiking, seeking new insights into the meaning of life while also extending theirs.

What is known about these early thinker walkers is not much; however, many of their thinking paths are still in use, like around Germany, Spain, and Greece. What we do know about serious hikers is that they testify to miraculous personal physical development. Many claim to have had some wonderful ideas about the tricky questions surrounding their personal life and its problems.

Thinking walks have many advantages. Walking through past memories and drifting into future possibilities are priceless experiences without the burdens of the present. Additionally, the experience is both physically and mentally relaxing. Here the mind does the walking and the body is stimulated, helping extend life's longevity.

Thought walkers are representative of us all in our most private moments. As with the swamp outlanders of our past, today every human has the capacity to take a "thought walk."

Biologists have a cute saying, "Ontogeny recapitulates phylogeny," meaning we all transit the various stages of life from where we began: ova and sperm to whatever stage we are now in, sometimes called human.

Thinking walkers are deeply engaged in multidimensional thoughts. They even try to sort out stuff like what is about to happen when we die or ascend – the latter still being a stretch. For sure they are never as they walk wired into Fox News or other emerging busted news reports. To these cerebral walking folks, there are only ephemeral questions, all without empirical answers.

Interestingly, almost all walkers will at one time or another slip into this stage of mental meandering. Therein lies our futures.

B. Walker Talkers

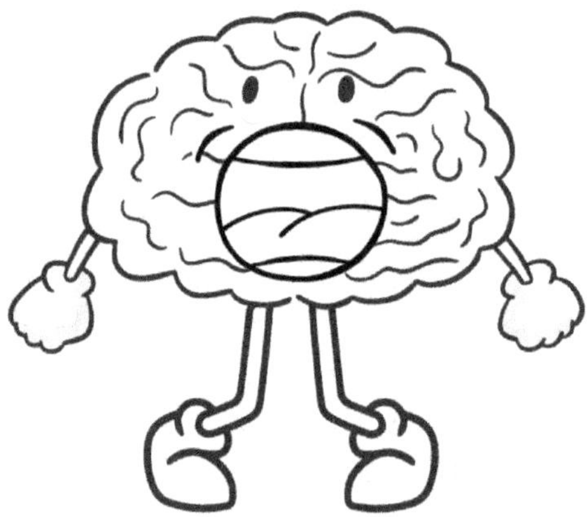

Walker talkers are sorta the species' alpha humans, no matter where you meet them. They have lots to say, and they also say lots. To what extent talking and walking correlate today is pretty much unknown. Benefits do include lung-throat exercise and sharing personal wisdom with all within earshot.

It is rumored, by some, that this walker talker category is more popular among the fairer sex. Probably because they know more and are generous in sharing. They engage in a sort of Ladies Aid Walk-a-thon. They all talk and walk at the same time and somehow seem to comprehend what they are all saying at the same time. Only quantum physics can explain this.

Males are very seldom seen simultaneously walking and talking in a bunch. For one thing, they are challenged at multitasking. Secondly, they would spill too much of their precious beer. Finally, perhaps they don't have that much to talk about or share.

Affiliations between mind, voice, jaw, and leg movements are being researched, e.g., does the walker's jaw drop as their right foot moves forward, or vice versa? And how do vocal sound waves relate to walkers' pace? The preference for the talking walkers may be related to one's zodiac orientation. Coil it be that talker walkers are an early sign of prophetic walking.

Another conundrum is the business of what walker talkers do with their arms while walking. Many seem to have these appendages flailing in sync with both their legs and mouths. They are a natural beauty to behold.

These gifted folks also tend to smile a lot, which energizes the people they meet on their paths. They have a unique capability to deflect whatever in hell you were thinking about and make you chuckle – at least privately – as you wonder what that was all about.

C. The Power Techie Walkers

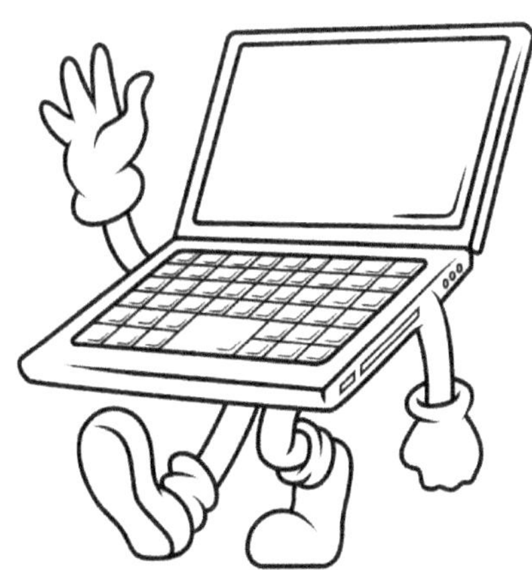

Look out! Power Walkers seem to be marching as if to make a statement, sometimes carrying a loaded briefcase (at least mentally), or swinging their arms like vanes on a Dutch windmill, grinding wheat. Their challenged hearts are beating like crazy to keep their run-amok body going. The benefit is that they may outlive all non-walkers.

Machine walkers represent the techie folks. They may indeed portend the future. Walking machines and measuring devices really excite current Luddites, who see them as uncivilized abominations. Well-meaning, perhaps even improving their personal health, machine walkers most certainly improve the bottom lines of technical industries and "fitness" peddlers.

These devices challenge the true meaning of walking, as machine walkers consume endless data about how fast they are going, how many steps they are taking, and how their heart and lungs correlate with their legs and feet. The machines distract walkers from being in touch with nature and instead draw their focus to cute silly dials, flashing garish lights, and clever videos, all designed to make you think you are walking. Many "treadmills" even set the machine walker in motion while watching television! Given, the machines do perhaps help your cardiovascular system, but at the cost of your mind. We now find this gimmicky walking and going nowhere is replacing what creative fish had in mind when leaving the swamp.

These avant guard fish had a new destination in mind – a new idea. An unknown idea, yet to be discovered. Can you imagine a fish swim machine? Even sexually excited salmon swimming upstream are going somewhere.

We see the machine walkers everywhere; even in the privacy of their homes, motels, and so called "sports centers." In these flashy centers the machine walker will freely share their gooey, smelly body fluids with everybody else – and feel good about it. Yuck, say the fish.

How in the world did humans, who naturally enjoy walking, mostly upright, come up with the wild idea to create these devices so they would not have to walk, just sit on a hard-butt bike and be entertained while simultaneously huffing and puffing? We are indeed an amazing species.

Machine walkers also have gimmicks that provide all kinds of essential(?) information, like how many calories per drop of sweat are you oozing per kilometer and at what rate? To do this, the machines weigh you before and after "the walk." Then timers kick in and you begin the ordeal. Machine walkers may believe it's a positive feature to be able to sit and watch on a monitor, "Sweaty Buddies in the Mountains." If that flick doesn't excite, they can try TV or read pulp magazines

Additionally, some machine walkers often have wires hanging everywhere and for sure a "phone" of some kind attached to a fist-like mic jammed in their face. And if they have a speaker-type phone, they now qualify as a power talker walker. They can't wait for a portable power printer. Since they may be stressed, and possessed, they need to walk off nervous energy. If you listen carefully you may often hear them yelling bars of Ole Johnny Phil Sousa's famous "El Capitan."

But by gawd they do show the world the power of walking. They will lose a pound or two, which they quickly replace by consuming super-charged lattes or ultra-diet sucrose energy bars, all washed down with Carlsberg Elephant beer. Power indeed.

Bystanders and sitters admire and envy their performance while simultaneously giving them a chuckle and wondering where and how they, too, could achieve this level of high-performance walking.

The past evolutionary fish, who got us going upright, would probably not be enthralled by this machine development. Just as swimming was no doubt boring for some fish, walking can become boring for some people. So now, just maybe, the next evolution following walking will be some kind of weird movement in space with a device that will enhance both swimming and walking, while doing neither – but going somewhere. Let us hope.

Juxtapose these power walkers with the thinker walkers. Draw your own conclusion – body, mind, or both.

D. Dressy Walkers

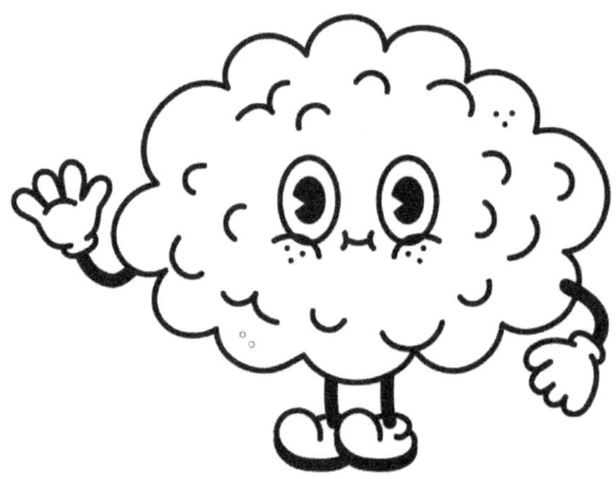

The earliest ex-swamp walkers had few dressy duds. Mostly gray, caked mud mixed with shiny green algae. But nowadays, people like to dress for any and all activities – and of course the fashion industry obliges.

Life's sole purpose for dressy walkers has nothing to do with philosophy or cardiovascular issues. It is all about what a walker wears. The hottest styles from global rag shops drive these walkers into hoofing it to the mall or spending hours on Amazon. Their ideal "end all" design is soooo tight-fitting that you can clearly detect hair images from their nether parts as they smugly strut along life's walking pathways. They do excite the like-minded walkers, as well as innocent bystanders, male and female, to ask them, "Where in the world did you get THAT outfit?" And of course, "What did you pay for it?"

Actually walking can be done in a variety of garments, as long as private parts aren't exposed or dragging. There seems to be a big unfulfilled market for creative walking clothing – you know, to keep your butt off the sidewalk and still look chic.

Not to belittle fashion in walking – it may often be the motivation for non-walkers to become walkers. Get out and strut your stuff. Follow the tradition of the Parisian flâneur, whose goal was to idly stroll about being sure to be seen.

This is a good place to start. But this is not the rationale for walking. Walking is for the interior, not the exterior.

An aside: Folks living and walking in warm climates are naturally scantily attired so as to keep cool. Walkers on Rio's Copacabana Beach save lots on clothing costs by being minimalists. Still, it's amazing how much design and expense can be attached to scanty scraps of Spandex. Need I say that this look is not for everyone?

E. Marathon Walkers

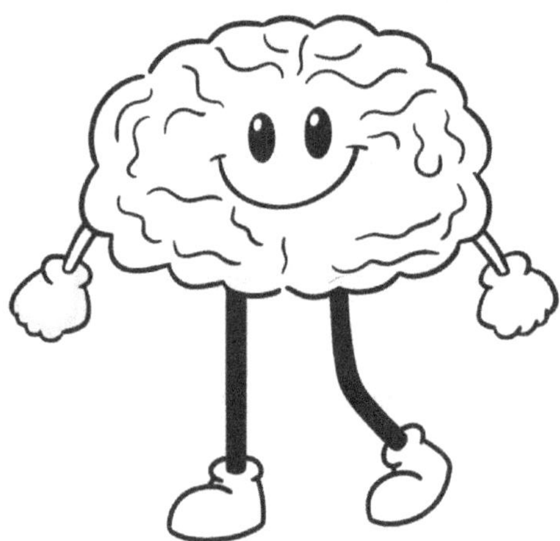

These venturesome creatures are superb walkers. While the rest of us don't have the gumption or predilection for giving up creature comforts, like toilets and downy beds, marathon walkers later become walking psychologists, handing out smiley face cards with office hours and shoe store locations.

Life's mission for some of them is to hike up really big hills, like Mt. Everest, of course with tireless Sherpas carrying their gear, selfie cameras, and beer. Others take long runs in Los Angeles and Boston on a regular basis. Some may do the California Johnny Muir trail before or during Happy Hour. They are the ultimate merit-badge walkers. After these momentous feats, these walkers deserve a happy moment to cool heels and trim bunions.

There are incredible walking/hiking routes all over the world. Some date back to pre-piston-locomotion time, which means that you can walk and walk and think and think. The claim is, such pilgrimages are exhilarating and beat riding a horse, a mule, or a llama.

For some unknown reason many European trails meander near or through vineyards. It is recognized that grapes are

Healthy, regardless of what you do with them before imbibing them.

F. Hippity-hop Walkers

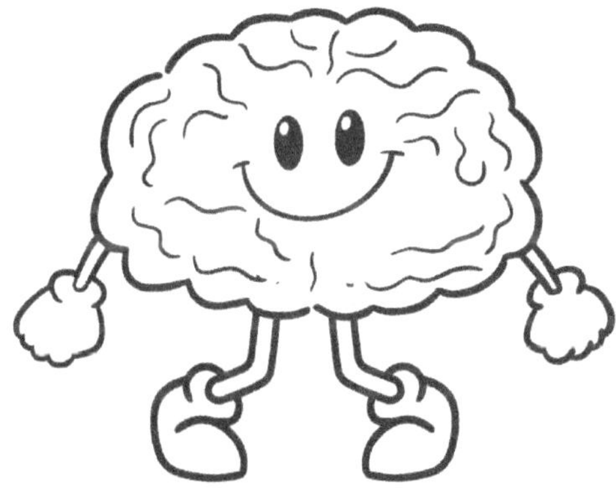

Walking erratically, stopping frequently, sometimes singing while taking in their surroundings are the hippity-hop walkers. Shaking hands and hugging appalled onlookers, they provide free entertainment for the observing bench sitters. They take time to smell the roses and chat with passersby who often are animal walkers.

From a health point of view, hippity-hop walkers are probably using more calories and flexing more body parts than other, more ordinary walkers. But you have to be careful walking near them – they might just end up in your arms. If they do smile at you, acknowledge them by smiling back, but be careful before giving them your cellphone number – unless your guest list is really short or you have many unused minutes on your contract.

Many in this category carry selfie supplies and will take pictures of everything along their path, of course featuring their smiley puss in front of everything. They are happy souls, enjoying creation and stimulating the rest of us. The more stoic walker types wish they could be this free and unfettered.

G. Yodel Walkers

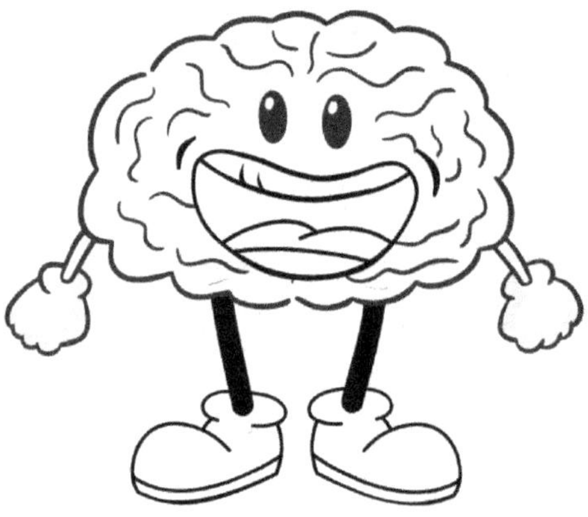

These are rare (thank god), but there are walkers who enjoy unrestrained, often off-key singing or sometimes simply cackling while taking an afternoon stroll before the bars get hopping. Often they seemingly expect a return echo, so when encountered you should give a simple but sincere smile and pick up your own pace so as to not break their spell or their anticipated return echo.

You may never know where in the universe these souls come from or are living, but for them it is good mental health that they are out walking and breathing fresh air. Many yodel walkers have been to the Rockies, Alps, or Himalayas, where they may have picked up this intriguing yodeling habit. The good news is there are no known serious acts of political unrest committed by these walking vocal enthusiasts. "The Hills are alive…"

Walking can be like taking a soft warm shower. It makes you want to sing about all the wonderful thoughts you had along the path – providing of course you can untangle the electronic devices distracting you from breaking news reports.

H. Collector Walkers

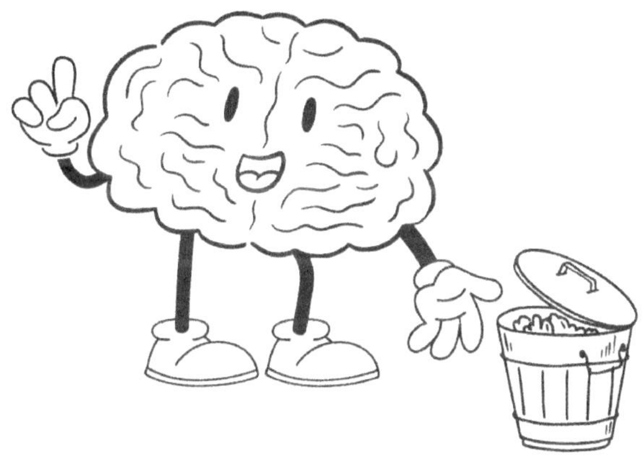

True heroes are these walkers. They remind you of seagulls who constantly and generously clean up polluted beaches -- polluted not by them, but by humans. Similarly, collector walkers scan the ground before them to find precious items that have been inadvertently lost or recklessly discarded. Some use high-tech metal detectors that are loaded with sensitive devices that screech in the walker's ears that riches are near.

The downside of looking down is they might run headlong into other walkers, big trees, or community-provided dumpsters.

These social-minded walkers help keep walkways clean and beautiful. If you try to tip them they often get upset, since they are the truly rich, at least in spirit, walkers.

Many of these community-minded collectors are also collecting experiences and memories of the "who in hell throws this stuff away?" Most likely the litterers are mere slobs, but perhaps some are folks wishing to relieve themselves of certain memories? What was the meaning of this discarded item?

These walkers, who not only keep walkways clean and nice, also preserve the memoirs of a discarded past. They are like waves that periodically cleanse and wash away the past.

I. Wheelie Walkers

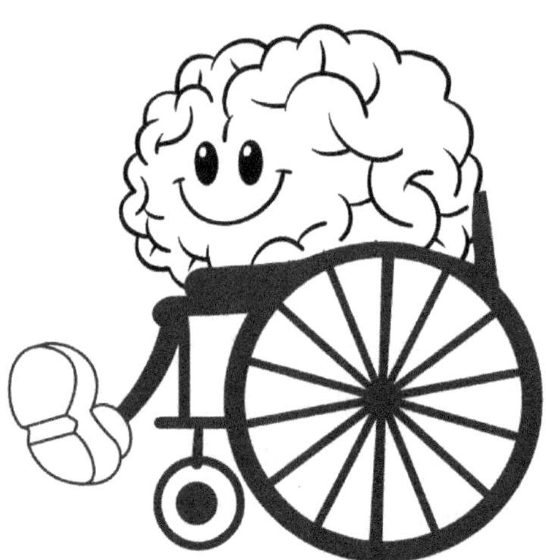

These are the venturesome walkers who have lost the physical capacity to walk and have a deeper perspective on the meaning and value of walking. They are not encumbered and valiantly demonstrate their independence as they wheel along.

The creators of these ersatz walking devices have opened doors to new vistas for those who, through heroism and/or bad luck, have lost the ability to put on shoes and take a hike. These bright, sensitive creators of "walker wheels" have helped wish-to-be walkers move from the impossible to the possible. Gallant behavior.

Some wheelie walkers are solo walkers. Others walk pushing very precious cargo, be it a kid or two in high-tech buggies or, in some cases, pampered animals who are either handicapped or overly indulged and wish they could chase the ever-present birds or other dogs.

One set is parents or surrogate parents, strolling with darlings who enjoy the rolling/rocking transition from their previous watery womb environment to future Wall Street boardrooms. Here walking/strolling is a serious, often paid-for business. We also see weekend strollers – modest parents whose darlings are destined to be engineers, teachers, and bricklayers and are momentarily bonding with their offspring, the meaning of their life. These folks truly tug at your heartstrings, having squirreled time from inane work to take a walk and momentarily experience a certain level of freedom and privacy.

J. Animal Walkers

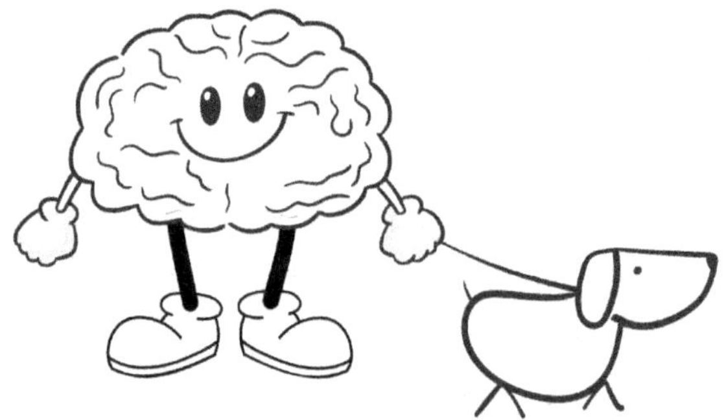

These walkers are blessed. They have the human decency to take otherwise-cooped-up animals for an airing and opportunities to pee and poop as their nature calls them. For a few precious moments these animals have all the natural dignities befitting their breed. They can smell, hear, and sense life in the "wild," be it Central Park or Rodeo Drive.

The humans at the other end of their leash are equally blessed. They, if properly trained, will pick up the animal's deposits and dispose of it to protect others from stepping in it.

Furthermore, human brains are engaged in a struggle with an animal that in most cases they can't control. Remember how General Patton had a rambunctious pitbull he dragged around during the Second Great War? Some comments were made that you could not tell them apart except for their number of legs. This is still true in many cases. Have you not noticed that dog food makers often make their products sound like top-of-the-line gourmet fare – fit for human consumption?

Any animal that encourages and assists humans to walk deserves credit. This of course means animals are responsible for the lengthening human life expectancies. Sadly, too often our life extenders are poorly treated, even abused.

Most often animal walkers are walking with dogs. Cats, kangaroos, and parrots are much too smart to willingly submit to the demeaning situation of being tied to a human being. Seeing cat owners trying to get putty-tat to go for a stroll clearly demonstrates that our mental machineries are different. One of these participants is clearly stupid. It may vary which one.

Animal walkers do not have the luxury of doing much thinking while walking. They are busily restraining their colleague, while mouthing all kinds of things, in whatever language they themselves understand. Needless to say most dogs don't speak human, but many do seem to pick up on what the leash-holder is trying to convey. Between their woofs and arfs, the dogs will also give looks back at the walker – like, "Get real, buddy, and stop your baby talk."

Dogs are constantly looking for spots to identify and claim as their territory. This activity is a constant distraction, which means the walker has little time to mentally commune with their natural surroundings. This is good, because now the walker is dutifully walking but not realizing it. One might say that walking dogs provides a narcotic numbing effect on the walker, many of whom do not relish the dog walking in the first place.

K. Comfy Walkers

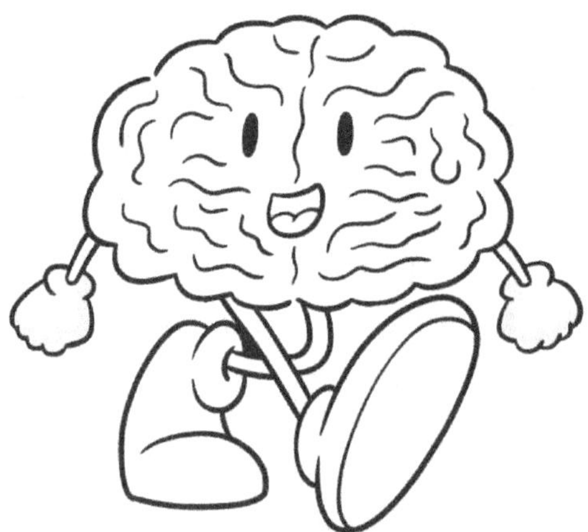

The rest of us can appreciate being the comfortable walker, especially since this category probably describes most of us. No particular reason for taking a walk – it just feels good. No need for tight-fitting derriere-revealing leggings or wide-brim hats with ludicrous decorations. Just whatever one happens to have on and is legal is sufficient.

These people may just want to walk off a fantastic, or bad, meal, get away from their cubby hole desk loaded with tasks that are anything but challenging, and stretch their cramped legs and befuddled minds. They have also been studying up on reports on the health benefits of walking.

Comfy walkers are simply reacting to unfulfilled mental and bodily issues or simple, everyday unfulfilled dreams. If and when they get a serious or depressing thought while walking, it is usually relieved by breaking wind, which quickly disburses in the open air. These walkers have everything to gain by taking a short hike.

Since we acknowledge that each human's mind is different, it is no wonder we all have a unique walking style – and maybe that is good. The key is to keep walking.

L. Marchers and Dancers

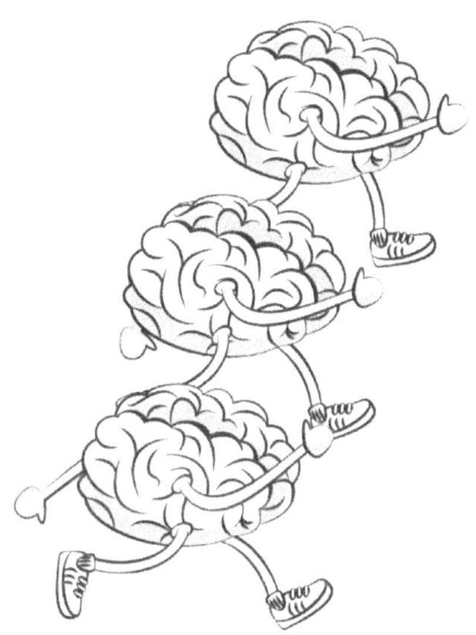

Marching and dancing – the last and most exciting walker category. The skills needed to be a marcher or dancer are many, beginning with the brain becoming disciplined. First, the marching brain must accept musical rhythms as instructions to be obeyed. Overlaid on the various musical beats come instructions on pace and direction of movement, coordination of orientation, and of arms and legs.

Then, most importantly for marching, the brain must fully obey the baton of a single leader. It is no wonder that marchers are the symbols of obedience, group power, and of course, fun

It is indeed an inspirational experience for marchers to collectively obey their brains and unite in orchestrating a plethora of legs to be in sync with each other and to the melodies of marching music.

For ballet, all body movements must be incredibly disciplined. Here it is not only arms and legs, but the entire body and mind that are controlled. For most other dancers, the legs will duly follow instructions, but in general the dancing body has more freedom of motion. .

The great news is that marchers and dancers alike will extend their lives, probably indefinitely, just like all who simply walk. The key is to keep moving.

Chapter Six

Reminiscing

These comments reflect wonderful memories and muddled thoughts about our species' past experiences and future possibilities. Trust me, you can only do this kind of thinking when walking and looking forward to happy hours.

Always remember: whenever you fish, for food or ideas, there is a history of previous folks/creatures who genetically got you where you are today. All over our world philosophical topics were and are discussed while walking rustic nature trails or polluted urban streets.

"Walk the Thought." should replace "Walk the Talk". After all, it is the brain that is in charge, not the talk.

What a great requirement for all politicians – insist, these sometimes dimwits, debate their thoughts while marching up and down the streets of Washington. May encourage them to stay on topic and be honest? If the streets of WDC don't do it, how about the Grand Canyon? Here they can yodel to their heart's content.

One has to wonder how many great/greatest ideas and creations were conceived while their creator was hiking as opposed to sitting at a desk pecking away with fingers.

Walking brings new visions and integrates them with memories of past experiences; creating innovative vistas and promises for the future. Remember, fish and frogs showed the way.

Another major walking benefit, solo walkers can safely admit to themselves their faults, misdeeds, sins, and mistakes. By confessing to yourself, you may even become honest with yourself – and all the while getting to live longer. What a system! Live longer, make more mistakes, then walk away and live even longer.

What helps make the walking experience so vibrant are the varieties of sensations walkers encounter, stimulating every sense organ – sight, smell, feel, sound – all being mixed in the mind.

The writer/walker of this book personally abhors electronic devices that detract from being alone with one's outer and inner self and thoughts. Earbuds, smart/dumb phones, tight-fitting blood-restricting clothes and the like, are viewed by this codger as distractions that rob walkers of their individuality, creativity, and enjoyment of life's many gifts. Instead of developing as a unique human entity, the "wired walkers" become simple responders to other prefabbed sensations. How tragic. How can these individuals ever make a personal contribution?

The author is trying to continue learning and appreciating the world about him – by himself – and urges you to do the same. Self-learning is facilitated and enhanced based on doing, observing, thinking and - walking.

SO DELAY YOUR DEATH NOW

WALK!

This has been a rambling narrative, from a somewhat dementing old curmudgeon, obtained from age, observations and reveries while taking daily walks along San Diego's Shelter Island, He still does this to stay alive and commune with his soulmate, Dixie Lee, who got him walking as she prepared to run the First Los Angeles First marathon.

THIS IS NOT THE END - FOLKS

JUST ANOTHER LIFE EXTENSION

-FOR WALKERS!